TRAPPED
INSIDE MYSELF

*My Journey to Freedom
from My Obesity Prison*

Sheila Howard

TRAPPED INSIDE MYSELF

My Journey to Freedom from My Obesity Prison

ISBN (978-0-692-19430-0)

Editor: Angela Edwards, Pearly Gates Publishing

Book Cover Graphics and Design: Innomark Group

Book Cover Design Creation: Sheila Howard

Photographer: Eugene Howard

Dedication

I dedicate this book to my loving husband who has been my strength and support from the beginning. Your love, prayers, and encouragement mean everything to me. Many times, I found myself procrastinating and even wanting to quit, but you encouraged me to keep going. Thank you for helping me to believe I could do this. Your actions are a true reflection of unconditional love. You are my best friend, and I know God placed you in my life.

I love you Eugene!

"No one can tell your story, so tell it yourself.
No one can write your story, so write it yourself."

Author Unknown

Contents

Acknowledgments

7

Special Thanks

8

Disclaimer

9

Introduction: Trapped

10

Chapter 1: The Beginning

14

Chapter 2: Mental, Physical, and Spiritual Struggles

23

Chapter 3: Defining Moments Defined

32

Chapter 4: Defining Moments Unveiled, 1-6

37

Chapter 5: Defining Moments Unveiled, 7-9

51

Chapter 6: Weight Loss Surgery: My Life-Saving Tool
75

Chapter 7: Change Your Mindset
81

Chapter 8: Short-Term Goals
84

Chapter 9: Proper Nutrition
88

Chapter 10: Move It to Lose It: Exercise
91

Chapter 11: The Soul Connection: Prayer
95

Chapter 12: Find Support
100

Chapter 13: Make Yourself a Priority
103

Chapter 14: Final Thoughts
106

References
111

Acknowledgments

Thank you, GOD, for freeing me and letting me Live!

To all my beautiful children and grandchildren who have never seen me as anything but Mama and Mima: Thank you for simply loving me for me. You have my heart.

To my mother, Joan Smith, who displayed a healthy lifestyle in front of me all of my life: I love you and thank you for being an *amazing* example!

To my best friends—*my girls*—who continued to show support when I was whining, crying, and at my wit's end: Thank you!

Bishop John Williams: Your spiritual guidance, encouragement, and *incredible* wisdom truly helped me grow and remain focused. Thank you!

LaToya Williams: Thank you for sharing your wealth of knowledge while guiding me through this process!

To my natural, church, and online/virtual families: I appreciate your incredible words of support that have enriched my life and kept me pushing.

Special Thanks

Cassidy T. Chapman, Reginald S. Chapman, Carma Chapman, Madelia Buford, Lisa Matlock, Della Irving, Rita Smith-Nickens, Don Smith, Delwann Shahid, Madeline Thomas, Denine Lowery, Barbara Askew, Bernardette Kilgore, DeLondra Smith, Pastor Jewell and Lady Kellie Jones, Zelda Neese, Tonya Moore, Naajma Moore, Stacey Williams, Mekal Clinton, Tara Williams, Sally McGregor, Brenda Hunt, and LaRhonda Brown.

You all have impacted my journey either by simply being there for me or by something impactful that you said or did. *You know what it was!* Thanks for standing by me and providing unconditional love, support, and encouragement. You all have my sincere love and appreciation!

Sheila

Disclaimer

This publication is a testimonial describing my personal experiences. These accounts are from my perspective, and from the best of my recollection.

My results are being shared as inspiration. I am not a doctor, dietician, or licensed medical professional. I do not claim to cure any condition, cause, or disease. You should always consult your physician for direction involving health, nutrition, and weight loss.

Sheila Howard

Introduction

Trapped

Many people have experienced moments in life when they have felt trapped. Perhaps you have felt trapped in a situation, relationship, job, or maybe even in your own mind. You may have struggled with making a choice or decision but felt as if there was an invisible barrier preventing you from moving forward. The possibilities are vast.

You look for a way out, but feel like you're walking in a maze. Deep down, you know that a way out exists but you keep running into obstacles, walls, and barricades.

In most cases, after thought, prayer, and time you managed to find your way to an escape route. Perhaps your condition changes, you transition out of that relationship, find a new job, or get your thoughts on track and move forward to life's next adventure.

Like many, after feeling trapped for some time, I eventually moved away from unhealthy relationships. I left unfulfilling jobs and adverse situations that were not conducive to my growth and well-being. But there was one prison in which I was trapped for many years. I simply could not free myself. I was trapped in my own body — trapped in morbid obesity. It felt as if the *real me* was somehow stuck inside of a large and sickly body — **trapped inside myself.**

I have always loved myself. Even though I did not like the package I lived in, I still loved the person within. Even with my obvious flaws and imperfections, I have always valued and appreciated the person God made me to be internally. I remained grateful and have always been happy with myself and sought to be better.

An analogy that describes my feelings is like living in a house you do not care for or in a neighborhood you do not prefer, but you still manage to take pride in where you are. You mow your lawn, plant flowers, trim the hedges and even wash the windows of your house. You are in a house you do not want to be in forever, but you still do everything in your ability to care for it while you are there. Meanwhile, you are still looking for a new home and neighborhood in which you would be more comfortable. You are constantly in search of the home that is better suited for your needs, health, and well-being. Sadly, I was very uncomfortable in my own "house" and sought a way to move to a better place. I wanted a place — a body — that I could call home.

I am sharing my story to spread hope. My prayer is that I inspire someone. This is a very challenging journey filled with numerous ups and downs. The downs often wear you out to the point where you feel like giving up. I want someone to say that because of something I said or did, they did not give up. Then, I will know my struggles were not in vain.

*"Many days, I looked in the mirror but did not recognize the reflection.
I was losing myself inside myself."*

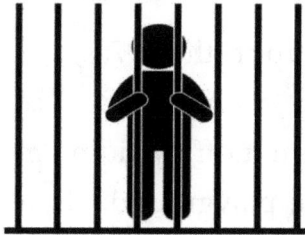

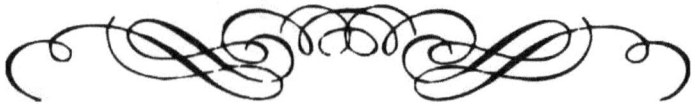

Chapter 1

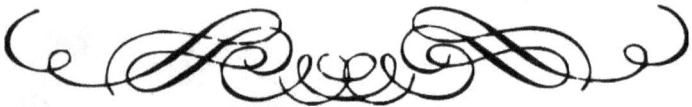

The Beginning

Growing up in the 1970s, I was a fairly active child. Like many young people, I could eat whatever I wanted and burn it off by riding my bike or playing hopscotch on the playground. I gave no thought to my body size or composition. Health and nutrition were not at the forefront of my mind. Being skinny was not intentional: it was automatic. I do not recall a single moment where I felt concerned about my weight. It was what it was — and that was it.

Other than a few isolated instances, I have never much dealt with low self-esteem issues. I have been blessed to come from a background of positive reinforcement from both my home environment and church community. I was also blessed with a certain degree of personal pride that motivated me to love and believe in myself regardless of my circumstances.

My weight issues began in my 20s as I began to gain and retain weight after two childbirths and also as a result of life in general. Over the years, I managed to get in some sporadic exercise with gym memberships, but I lacked consistency. Between the ages of 20 and 45, I gradually piled on 225 pounds. By the time I was 45 years old, my youthful, lean, 125-pound body had grown to an unhealthy and life-threatening 350 pounds. I was classified as morbidly obese.

While morbid obesity was the state that I was very uncomfortable in, I still tried to be the best me that I could be—even within the confines of my painful prison. This something for which I will always be grateful. Without faith and some degree of self-love, the road to improvement and progress is extremely challenging. Even with a reasonable degree of self-esteem, this extreme level of change took its toll.

There I was, trapped in a painful shell, running aimlessly around a maze of weight loss options. I was looking for an escape route but found myself crashing into painful brick walls. The person I wanted to be was getting more and more buried, and I was terrified that I would be trapped in that prison forever. Unable to live life to my fullest potential because of physical challenges and continually dealing with the fear of judgment and rejection, I was losing myself inside myself.

We have all seen those television commercials where someone says they have tried all the different diets, only to have short-term or minimal success, and then regain the weight plus some. Well, I could have easily been one of those folks. While others whom I knew personally were having success with those diets, I always failed. For some reason, my body did not respond positively. I could not understand why.

In my desperation, I went in search of a prescription weight loss method and was told about a weight loss pill that would practically melt the fat away. Word was spreading about a very popular physician known around town as "That Diet Doctor." Word on the street was "That Diet Doctor" would get you together! Well, they didn't have to tell me twice!

I made an appointment with him to find out if he would treat me. He acquired my health history, administered a quick exam, and wrote me a prescription for the weight loss medicine and a diuretic to help with my obvious water retention issues.

The doctor monitored my weight loss progress on a weekly basis. Even though the pills gave me jitters, they helped me lose some weight. Over the course of just a few months, I managed to lose a little greater than 50 pounds! I thought I had hit the jackpot! I traded my size 18 jeans for a size 14, and you couldn't tell be a thing, Jack! But while I was ecstatic about the weight loss, deep down on the inside, I knew I couldn't continue to take pills forever. This antidote was too good to be *true*.

Eventually, I found it more and more difficult to get the prescription for the diet pills filled. Most pharmacies did not carry the medication and, as if they were somehow offended, many drug stores would practically throw the prescription back to me after reading the medication's name. Of course, this made me suspicious, and I decided that perhaps I should do some research on the drug. But before I even had a chance, I saw a news story about the dangers of this popular diet pill. It was suspected of causing heart problems, and many doctors and pharmacies chose to discontinue its use. It got to the point where I could hardly turn on the news and not hear a negative story about the drug. It was back to the drawing board for me. I regained the 50 pounds — and then some.

I joined numerous weight loss support groups, looking for answers and direction. Although these groups provided some useful knowledge and meal plans, I achieved minimal success. I also participated in weight loss challenges at my workplace. I joined forces with coworkers that were also striving for healthier lives. We set a dollar amount and contributed to a pot on a weekly basis. The money served as an incentive. The grand prize was to be awarded to the person who lost the most weight in a particular timespan. As motivating as this experience was, and as hard as I tried, I lost. I did not lose any significant weight; just money. All of my unfruitful efforts made me sad and discouraged.

Since diets alone were not working for me, I decided to begin a rigorous exercise regimen. Even though I had worked out here and there, I knew that I needed to become consistent. I hired a phenomenal personal trainer who was also a professional bodybuilder and competitor. She was cut up! She had an amazing physique and embodied my desired look. I found her to be very encouraging and a great fit for me. Having a personal trainer stretched my budget a bit but I needed the guidance, so I deemed the expense worth it.

My trainer wrote me out a meal plan and instructed me to log every morsel of food I ate daily. I did so—religiously. This helped me discover just how well a food log will open your eyes to your actual consumption habits.

During this time, Tae Bo exercise videos were popular fitness tools. In addition to her own methods, my trainer used the videos during our indoor training sessions. I oddly enjoyed every painful moment! I felt an oxymoronic feeling of joy *and* pain that was very satisfying. I always felt exhilarated after training.

Once again, after months of strict training and diet, my body still looked the same. I had more energy and stamina, but my body held on to the weight for dear life. I was baffled. I could not understand why I was failing yet again. I got so discouraged that I decided to discontinue the workout sessions. When I broke the news to my trainer, she urged me not to give up. Unfortunately, I felt hopeless and was inconsolable. She went as far as to offer to train me at no cost if I just did not quit. But sadly, I could no longer mentally handle working so hard without seeing results. It had yet to be confirmed, but it was at this moment I *knew* there had to be something medically wrong with me.

In this book, I share many of the experiences that led me to make one of the most significant decisions of my life: to explore a surgical weight loss option. My story is just that—*my story* and *my testimony*. While I make no apologies for my choices, I realize there is no "one size fits all" health and weight loss regimen. I clearly understand that one thing may work great for one, but may not be ideal for another.

At the moment that they were happening, many of the accounts I write about here did not feel great. I *now* admit that some of them have some degree of humor attached. In retrospect, I have embraced that fact that some of my most challenging and even painful moments contained comical portions. I have chosen to see the humor in my instances as opposed to only seeing the pain. This is a viewpoint that I cherish. I appreciate that my story has joy and pain, sunshine and rain. I want to share my story in such a way that my readers will relate to more than just the struggle. It is my desire that they also are entertained and enlightened. I truly want to convey to anyone struggling with any situation (not just weight-related) that with faith *and works*, there is hope.

"Everyone has struggles, but many can be masked. Obesity cannot be hidden, therefore allowing others the opportunity to weigh in with their opinions and judgments. Oh, how I longed for an invisible struggle."

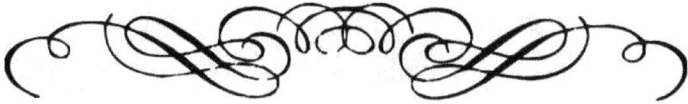

Chapter 2

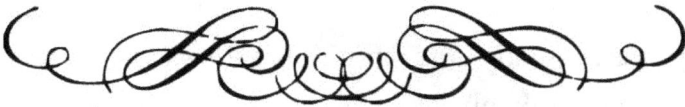

Mental, Physical, and Spiritual Struggles

In one way or another, my condition affected all facets of my life. My mental, physical, and spiritual lives were affected. For me, the three components were intertwined, and I could not fully and successfully progress without addressing all three of these crucial mechanisms.

Mental Struggle:

I mentally struggled with questions as to why—even after trying so hard to fight this condition—I was still trapped? Why—after the workouts, gym memberships, personal trainer, medical tests, diet pills, weight loss shakes, dietary food plans, self-help books, and videos—was I still trapped?

As an obese person, I often wondered if I was judged. There is an assumption that overweight people are greedy and lazy. I have found it rare for people to think obesity can be linked to something medical. I believe the most popular consensus is that obesity is strictly a condition reserved for gluttonous and slothful people. While I admit I could have done a better job in learning how to improve my general health, there was a limit to what I could achieve without help. That was something I really did not grasp at the time. The continued fight-and-fail roller coaster ride definitely took its toll on me mentally. As a person with a reasonable degree of self-confidence, constant failure in this fight made me feel—quite literally—like a big, fat loser.

I have heard the expression "dumb jock" all my life, but I have always been impressed with athletes. I have always been envious of the fact that they could control their bodies. There is no way you can be dumb and achieve some of the incredible things that athletes accomplish. If an athlete chooses to run, they run. If they decide they want to jump hurdles, they jump. Whether for personal pleasure or competitively, athletes set physical goals, make up their minds, train their bodies and their bodies respond accordingly.

I understood the concept of making up my mind and doing what was necessary for my body to line up with it. However, it still did not work for me. I could never understand why I could not make my body do what I wanted it to do. It is mental anguish to be able to control many areas of your life but not control the very body in which you live.

Spiritual Struggle:

One of the most difficult and challenging aspects of my time spent obese was the spiritual struggle I endured. As a believer in God and a believer that He can do anything but fail, I struggled to understand how I continued to fail — even at times when my faith was at its peak. I understood that "faith without works was dead," so, with that understanding, I did what I thought to be my due diligence — my "works." I looked for relief from my situation and was willing to make changes.

There were many times when I prayed and fasted for God to deliver me from my obesity. Many of my prayers for other things were granted (all of which I'm eternally grateful), but my prayer for physical healing seemed to be ignored. At the time, I had no idea there was a purpose for my pain. I didn't realize that my test was leading me into my testimony.

My favorite Bible passage is Philippians 4:13 which reads: "*I can do all things through Christ who strengthens me.*" This is my go-to scripture whenever I am dealing with something or struggling to accomplish a particular goal. I have always been able to quote the scripture and use it as a motivational tool to move me to the next level. I have those words hidden in my heart and on the tip of my tongue. However, in my fight for freedom from my morbid obesity prison, I could not do it. This was a major conflict for me. I was constantly *saying,* "I can do all things through Christ who strengthens me," yet I did not feel strengthened. I could not do this one thing that I so desperately wanted. My faith was seriously tested.

Physical Struggle:

Everyone has struggles. No one is exempt from issues, whether mentally or physically. However, some issues can be masked. There are some things individuals deal with that people in the general population would never guess or pick up on. Although they may be serious, certain issues can remain private. This allows the person the luxury to fight through their problems without the judgment of others. Unless they share, others will not have the opportunity to weigh in with their opinions.

Obesity cannot be hidden. Even with beautiful clothes, stylish hairdos, and makeup, my obesity was evident. I often wished I could trade it for an invisible struggle. But what others did not see, was the incredible amount of physical pain in which I was living. I believe that common sense tells people that obesity comes with some physical discomfort; however, I do not know if others truly understand the amount of physical pain that comes with carrying extra weight. Being obese for an extended period of time—in my case, almost two decades—has major consequences. My body suffered tremendously.

I tried very hard to mask the degree of pain I was actually living with. I was in constant pain both while awake and while I was sleeping. It seemed as if there was no way to escape. I shared my truth with my husband (constantly) and a few besties, yet I chose not to reveal it to the masses. I am not even certain my children realized the actual degree of pain I was in. I did not want to worry or burden them with my woes.

I was diagnosed with Arthritis, High Blood Pressure, High Cholesterol, and Plantar Fasciitis (which led to three foot surgeries). I was suffering from incredible joint pain, fatigue, back pain, incontinence, insomnia, and bone pain. I was always cold, endured short-windedness, and could barely walk. Simple things like walking through the mall or climbing a flight of stairs resulted in a great deal of discomfort. Whenever possible, I tried to avoid those activities. Avoiding physical activity did nothing but contribute to my primarily sedentary lifestyle. I had the desire to participate in regular physical activity, but other than swimming, practically everything else increased my level of pain. Being trapped in that condition took a toll on my body.

I have always wanted to act in stage plays. For years, I allowed my shyness and weight issues to hold me back. When I finally got up the courage to audition and participate in a production, I was blessed to land the role of a grandmother. The director allowed me to name my character, and I became "Mother Crenshaw." Even though taking on this acting role was a leap of faith and a blessing for me, I knew my participation would come with some challenges.

During the first rehearsal, I could barely stand until the end. The pains in my legs and feet were overwhelming. Afterward, I asked the director if I could get a cane to make my character look more aged. He agreed, and I went to the drug store and bought a nice silver cane. The cane definitely fit into my costume, but secretly, I also needed to use the cane to help me stand for the rehearsals and final production. Walking and standing were so painful for me that I seriously thought about using the cane in my real-life activities. I consider this one of the lowest points of my journey.

*"I longed to get to the good part:
the physical version of the wonderful,
chewy, chocolate-flavored Tootsie Pop
center. But unlike the owl in the
commercial, there were no shortcuts."*

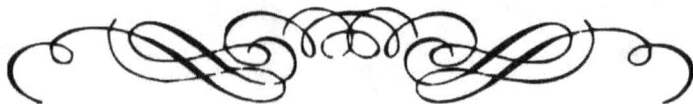

Chapter 3

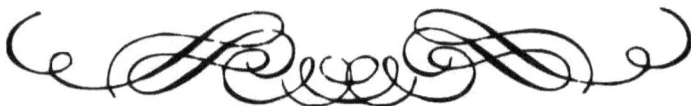

Defining Moments Defined

Although I knew I needed to do something different (perhaps drastic) to free myself, I clung to some fantasy hope that one day the weight would just fall off. I hoped that one of the popular diets would be "the one" that would work for me and my life would be permanently changed! While I waited for this saving grace, I had many defining moments that shouted to me that I needed to seek out help.

The dictionary expresses a "Defining Moment" as *"the time that shows very clearly what something is really about."* In most cases, when people experience a *defining moment*, the light comes on such as it should, and a significant or perhaps even life-changing action soon follows. In a perfect world, when we are shown very clearly what something is really about, we accept our truth or implement changes and move forward. This sounds so simple. Perhaps with many situations, it is just that simple.

That is the beauty of a defining moment. We receive eye-opening clarity or confirmation. Now, what if you receive a defining moment, recognize it, and make some degree of an effort to change but fail? What if you receive several defining moments, yet find yourself still trapped in the same predicament?

As a child, one of my favorite television commercials was a Tootsie Pop ad. A kid asks an owl, "How many licks does it take to get to the Tootsie Roll center of a Tootsie Pop?" Instead of slowly licking the candy, Mr. Owl (as he was cleverly called) prematurely bit through the outer candy shell to get to the delicious center. It is easy to be impatient when you know there is a delightful treat in store!

Really, how many licks *does* it take to get to the Tootsie Roll center of a Tootsie Pop? Mr. Owl said three, but it actually takes 364 licks (Yes, I googled it!) to get to the wonderful, chewy, chocolate-flavored center of a Tootsie Pop. The fruity candy coat is nice, but the center is the *good part*! In my adult life, as a member of the morbidly obese community, I received many defining moments that *should* have led me to do something drastic to better my life and health. Now, don't get me wrong: Many honest efforts were made to transform my ever-growing body into the trimmed, toned, muscular, and healthy woman I pictured in my mind. My efforts proved unfruitful.

Daily, I longed to get to the *good part*. I desperately desired to get to the physical version of my wonderful, chewy, chocolate-flavored Tootsie Pop center. Unlike the owl in the commercial, there were no such shortcuts. I will let you in on some of the moments that served as my wake-up calls. Those moments eventually led me to the Tootsie Roll center of my Tootsie Pop. They also led me to the restoration of my health and newfound, fantastic quality of life!

With both humility and pride, allow me to share some of the steps I took that led to the transformation of my 50-year-old, practically immobile, pain-stricken 350-pound body into the much healthier and leaner 186-pound body that I gratefully live in today.

"The fact that I awakened is far more important than how many wake-up calls it took. Woke is woke."

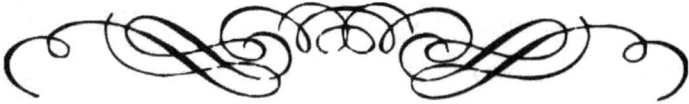

Chapter 4

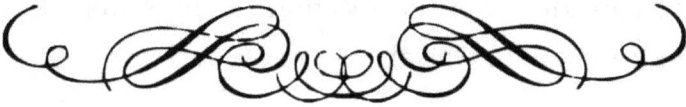

Defining Moments Unveiled
1-5

Defining Moment #1: The day I almost died at Comerica Park — or at least I thought.

A co-worker had extra tickets to the ballpark and offered them to me. I happily accepted the tickets, as I had never been to the newly-built Detroit Comerica Park. I was not a true-blue baseball fan, but I was still excited to get out, mingle, and do a little sightseeing in my beautiful city.

I was not in denial, but it was like I would somehow forget I was morbidly obese. I accepted and embraced social invitations. How could I forget that something as simple as a trip to the ballpark for most could be potentially traumatic for me? Parking and walking to enter the ballpark was one thing; what I didn't consider was the location of the seats. Little did I know what I was about to face.

We took the long haul up to the top level where our seats were located. I could barely maneuver the short steps. They seemed to go on forever. With every step I took, my heart was racing as if it was trying to beat its way out of my chest. What was I thinking? Why would I voluntarily put myself through this anguish? I seriously thought I would black out. It felt like it took three days to get to the very top row of Section 300 where our seats were located. I felt a smidgen of relief that I had at least made it to my seat.

The struggle was not over, though. No ma'am; no sir. Again, I had not thought this thing through. I had not thought about how small the seats would be in the ballpark. It is probably not the case, but it feels like venue seats are being made smaller and smaller. I was definitely getting bigger and bigger. Public seating is not accommodating to the obese community. I managed to wedge my whole self into the very hard, non-giving, metal ballpark seat.

I was now enduring shortness of breath, shooting pains in my feet, and pain in my throbbing chest. There was excruciating pain around my hips as they begrudgingly pushed themselves into the unwelcoming metal. My heart was beating so fast and hard, I literally thought I would die at Comerica Park. My mind was racing as I pictured the EMS running up the stairs with a stretcher (or two) to haul the morbidly obese black lady from the top level. I envisioned them trying to take me down, but with my body being so heavy, I would more than likely be dragged from step to step. Bloomp, bloomp, would be the sound of my backside as it hit and scraped each stair — and I would be mortified, were it not for me being dead.

I pictured the story headline in the Detroit News: "*Obese Woman Perishes after suffering Heart Attack at Comerica Park.*" The tragic story would be shared and re-shared on social media. Maybe it would even go viral. My mind and heart were racing. This was *not* where I wanted to die. This was not *how* I wanted to die. I did not *want* to die! I mean, if you are *going* to die, should not it at *least* be doing something you enjoy? I should have been dying on a dance floor or beach. I know I cannot choose how I go, but this certainly was not how I wanted to be remembered.

For about 15 minutes, my heart pounded against my chest as I contemplated telling my husband to call 911. It was arguably the scariest 15 minutes of my life. Eventually, my heart rate came down, and I realized I would live another day. Then, I was able to focus on the horrible pain of the metal seat digging into my hips and back as I pretended to enjoy the baseball game.

Defining Moment #2: Chairs

When most people sit down, they do so with little to no thought. Sitting is second-nature to the general public. Going to restaurants and sitting in a booth is another common practice for many. You have a seat and proceed to order your food without a single thought about the seat in which you are sitting. Well, as a morbidly obese person, sitting in chairs and booths were some of my most terrifying experiences. I lived with the constant fear of not fitting into a booth or on a chair. I was even afraid of having a chair break from my heavy weight.

Imagine how scary it is to be fearful of such a common, everyday practice. Before entering a restaurant, I experienced incredible anxiety and fear. What kind of chairs do they have? If the chairs have arms, will I fit? How close is the booth seat to the table? Will people stare at me as I wedge into the seat? My head would swim with questions as I approached the table. I had (for the most part) mastered the art of pretending there was no issue because I did not want to distress my dinner companions. Sometimes, I wanted to vent my pain, but I noticed how uncomfortable it made others feel. Only those closest to me were aware of the fear I was experiencing. They did not truly know the actual level of my distress, though.

It was a fear that began from the moment I accepted the dining date. It continued to increase while I prepared to go out. It was further magnified as I entered the restaurant and approached the table. To avoid this anxiety altogether, I was often tempted to decline social engagements.

The combination of my love and zeal for social interaction and my drive to fight kept me pressing forward. I was a fighter and refused to give in to my situation. Even while knowing I could possibly spend the next hour in discomfort and pain, I pressed on. Knowing that my heaving chest could either be painfully smashed between the booth and table or literally end up resting *on* the table, I still pressed on.

The average person has no reason to give thought to intricate details such as seating. As a morbidly obese person, it was always in my best interest to plan ahead — if possible. I did not want to find myself in an uncomfortable, painful, or embarrassing situation. Unfortunately, life doesn't always go as planned or even allow you the opportunity to plan.

At around 280 pounds, I learned that I could not trust chairs. One beautiful summer day, I sat down on a swinging bench with my husband. We were on my aunt's porch. Even though I hesitated to sit, I took a chance. There we sat, chatting and enjoying the beautiful weather. Just when I thought I was in the clear and that the swing was on my side, it happened: I heard clank-clank...BOOM!

My side of the swing crashed to the ground, and my husband slid down onto me like two dominoes falling. My body weight was far too great for the swing. To say I was mortified would be an understatement. My husband tried to console me by saying, "The bench was already unsteady." Even if that were so, I was inconsolable. I managed to withhold my tears for the moment, but I was crushed. Sadly, even to this day (and 162 pounds lighter), I still find myself doing a chair test. I am always checking to ensure my weight will be supported. I am honestly uncertain that I will ever be completely rid of that impulse.

Defining Moment #3: Fat-Shaming

I have been blessed with some beautiful friends who are more like sisters. Two of my best friends and I decided to celebrate our sisterhood with a 10-year friendship getaway in Chicago. We packed our bags and headed for our getaway full of expectations of laughter, new experiences, and lifelong memories. We enjoyed a beautiful downtown Chicago hotel suite full of classic comfort. Besides shopping, our itinerary included a friendship gift exchange and dining at some of the city's well-known and highly-rated restaurants. On the list was a popular breakfast spot which was nearby. We excitedly ventured over. Despite the crowd and long line, we waited patiently to be seated. We watched others who arrived after us be seated before us. Amongst ourselves, we began to question why our wait was so extensive. Yes, even though it was a busy Saturday morning, our wait had been extreme.

After holding my tongue for a while, I let my sisters in on the reason for the wait. I had already noticed how the greeter looked at me with disdain. He scanned me up and down and gave me *the look.* I let my friends know this was a classic case of fat-shaming. I enlightened them to the fact that we were not being seated because of my size. I felt humiliated.

My wonderful friends (who always have my back) seemed to struggle with believing I was the cause of our extended wait. Their kindheartedness was endearing, but not my reality. We saw several people seated in open booths, while we stood around waiting. Eventually, the greeter came closer, and we asked why we were waiting so long. He said he thought we would be happy that he was *trying* to seat us in a place that would be "more comfortable for our situation." He was referring to him finding a table that would accommodate the fat lady, as opposed to a booth that he thought I would not be able to fit into.

The look on my friends' faces saddened me. My truth became apparent. Did this greeter think he was doing me a favor? I told him we would be fine in a booth and to go ahead and seat us. As he guided us to an open booth, he appeared to scoff as if to say, "Good luck." Thankfully, the booth was roomy. I was able to slide into it easily and without making a scene.

Unfortunately, my breakfast was ruined. I attempted to make small talk with my friends about other subject matter, but my fat-shaming experience dominated my thoughts. I felt extremely embarrassed. Although I did not allow it to ruin the trip for me completely, it absolutely stood out as a mortifying experience. Even though I felt terrible, it felt worse knowing I put my friends in an uncomfortable situation. This was yet another instance that made me contemplate discontinuance of public social interaction.

Defining Moment #4: Judgment and Assumptions

As with most people, some of the best moments with my family and friends are spent at the dinner table. Whether it is at home or in a restaurant, many special moments are built around meals or even just a cup of coffee. So, when my oldest friend called and suggested we meet for a bite to eat, I happily agreed. I relished any opportunity to share bonding moments with my sisters.

She had been craving a banana split and suggested we meet at a local big chain restaurant. On that day, in walked my beautiful friend who, over the years, maintained her slender, girlish figure. Whether her maintenance was due to genetics, great diet choices, or a combination of the two, it was something I have always admired. The hostess took our order. My friend ordered her banana split to her liking, and I ordered a salad with blue cheese dressing on the side.

The person who brought our food out was not the same person who had taken our orders. When the woman came out with the salad and the banana split, without hesitation, she sat the banana split in front of me and the salad in front of my friend. My friend quickly corrected her and let her know that the ice cream belonged to her. As she sized the two of us up, the waitress stated (clearly and without thinking) that she would have thought it would have been the other way around. She switched the dishes and placed the salad in front of me and the banana split in front of my friend.

As always, I did my best to mask my true feelings. I had feelings of embarrassment and anger as

I was, once again, judged by my size. The woman quickly assumed the smaller person was going to eat the salad and the obese person would (apparently) be eating the ice cream. This is one of the typical judgments that obese people endure on a regular basis. Furthermore, there's nothing wrong with an obese person enjoying an ice cream treat. That was not the issue. The issue was being judged without having any information. How could one be so bold as to rudely vocalize their assumption to customers?

Defining Moment #5: Seatbelts

Thank God for seatbelts. As inconvenient as they sometimes feel, seatbelt use is not only the law but is also potentially life-saving. Even before seatbelt use became law, I took no issue in wearing my seatbelt on my own. I had heard of drivers and passengers who were tragically ejected from their vehicles and suffered greatly—some even fatally. That was something I did not want to experience. Sadly, seatbelts can be very uncomfortable for an obese individual. Many vehicles and seatbelts are not made to accommodate larger people.

In 2014, Reuters Health reported that obese drivers may be at a much higher risk of a fatality in a car crash than normal-weight drivers due to frequently opting not to use their seatbelts. Heavier people often struggle to fasten their seatbelt. This was definitely the case for me. Additionally, the top portion of the belt would slide over my heaving chest and practically wrap around my neck. The belt often rubbed and chaffed my neck. I tried seatbelt extenders, but they always slid off. Many times, I have buckled up but feared the belt would either bruise or slice my neck. I even had terrifying thoughts of being decapitated after being in a crash as the belt actually did its job of holding me in place. Imagine driving every day with this constant fear. It was part of my reality.

*"Change happens when
the pain of staying the same is
greater than the pain of change."*

- Tony Robbins -

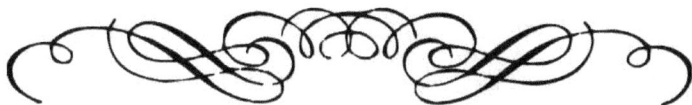

Chapter 5

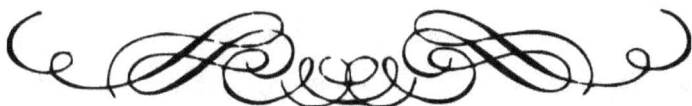

Defining Moments Unveiled
6-9

Defining Moment #6: Breast Cancer Biopsy

According to the National Cancer Institute, among women ages 40 - 50, African-American women have a higher incidence of breast cancer than any other race. Also, people who are obese have a higher likelihood of being diagnosed with cancer.

As an obese African-American woman within this age range with a family history of breast cancer, I have always taken my annual screening very seriously. After a mammogram, I would usually get a phone call or letter stating there we no signs of cancer followed by a standard closing that stated, "See you next year!"

In 2012, I received a call stating that my x-ray needed to be repeated due to a suspicious speck. A calcium deposit was suspected, but additional tests were needed for confirmation and to rule out cancer. Even after the second test, the results necessitated further clarification. I was scheduled for a large core biopsy. This test requires the patient to lie face down on a table so that a tissue sample can be collected.

While I consider myself a person of faith, and I knew that "God had not given me the spirit of fear," my human side was nervous. Even so, I scheduled the appointment. When I arrived at the hospital, the staff realized I was a heavy person and inquired about my weight. I was around 335 pounds at the time. I was well over the weight limitation of the biopsy table. I'm still not sure why this was not communicated to the staff in advance.

The staff scuffled around trying to figure out how to service me. On top of the nervousness I felt about possibly having breast cancer, I had to deal with the embarrassment of being too large for medical equipment. I was a combination of both fearful and ashamed. My God; even with all the remarkable advances in today's technology, the medical field was not prepared to accommodate my situation.

The surgeon was called in, and she somehow figured out a way for me to position myself and manipulate the machine to get the biopsy done. I was positioned almost upside down, and the experience graduated from incredibly uncomfortable to painful. The concerned staff constantly asked if I was okay and I continuously replied that I was fine. After all, it was my fault that I was heavy, not theirs. I had to deal with the consequences. As usual, although I was terrified on the inside, I managed to keep a calm, cool front.

Then, something amazing happened. When the ordeal was over, the surgeon hugged me, told me she would agree with me in prayer, and assured me that I would be fine. She was a woman of science *and* a woman of faith. I broke down and sobbed in her arms.

Thankfully, the tests came back with no signs of cancer! I was relieved, but I could not help but wonder if I would be back in this situation the following year. I was afraid that remaining trapped in my overweight state would continue to make me a likely candidate for a major illness like cancer. My relief was short-lived.

Defining Moment #7: Hypothyroidism

Over the years, my extreme weight gain has been (for the most part) unexplainable. Of course, my lack of physical movement and less than great dietary choices contributed to my size, but it still didn't explain the rapid weight gain and the inability to lose weight, even with diet and exercise.

On several occasions, I sought medical attention to help me understand why my body continued to grow and (even stranger) why my body resisted weight loss efforts. The tests continued to come back showing that all my functions were normal. Eventually, one doctor decided to check my thyroid. The tests indicated that my thyroid was functioning normally but the symptoms of a malfunctioning thyroid yet persisted.

A few more years went by where I continued to deal with my issues. I started seeing a new Primary Care Physician whom I found to be very attentive and thorough. After monitoring me, she noticed symptoms of a very slow metabolism function. She also saw signs of a possible goiter in my neck. She decided to check my thyroid functions, as she suspected possible thyroid problems. She sent me to a specialist—a noted Endocrinologist—who had the same suspicions. I couldn't see it, but with his trained eye, he could see the goiter starting to protrude from my neck. He sent me for a Fine Needle Biopsy and an Ultrasound. The tests confirmed there was a very large goiter and two benign nodules on my thyroid. Then, I was officially diagnosed with Hypothyroidism.

Hypothyroidism is an underactive thyroid gland that cannot keep the body running normally. The body's processes slow down as the metabolism slows down. Common symptoms of hypothyroidism are obesity, fatigue, hair loss, joint and muscle pain, and sensitivity to cold. This illness fosters unexplained weight gain and impedes weight loss. I was experiencing all of these symptoms.

Even though I was not happy about the diagnosis, I was somewhat relieved. While my lifestyle could have been better, I never believed my diet choices alone matched up to my severe weight gain. At least now I had an explanation for the way I was feeling. In many ways, this diagnosis was the first step into a glimpse of **hope.**

In 2007, after several biopsies and two years of monitoring my condition, my doctor finally decided to perform a thyroidectomy. The surgery was to remove my large, underactive thyroid which was now causing me to choke. Following surgery, my doctor said the removal had been a good call, as my thyroid was three times the size of a normal thyroid. He remarked that he had never seen one as large as mine. I was placed on thyroid replacement medication to help regulate my levels and informed I would have to take those pills for the rest of my life. I secretly hoped my new medication would also help my weight to decline.

Defining Moment #8: My Doctor yelled at me, "The Final Straw!"

I had a remarkable Primary Care Physician. Not only did she examine me, but she also spent time talking to me and trying to help me resolve my physical issues. Over the years, she guided me through a diet and exercise regimen in hopes of alleviating pain and lowering my weight. No matter how devoted I was, I only received minimal results. My doctor witnessed my genuine efforts. It was evident to me that she wanted to help me become free from this entrapment.

She would regularly mention weight loss surgery as a possible option. Each time she brought it up, I would decline the very idea. Even though I knew a few people who had gone down that road and had some success, I considered that option drastic and chose to keep trying to lose the weight "on my own."

During one particular doctor's appointment, she suggested I attend a weight loss surgery consultation. I had grown tired of hearing about weight loss surgery at practically every doctor's appointment (appointments that were, by the way, increasing in frequency). I kindly and respectfully asked my doctor to never bring up the subject to me again. I truly believed that if I kept trying, I could lose the weight on my own — you know: "the natural way." My doctor obliged me and agreed to let the subject rest.

In 2011, I went to one of my many doctors' appointments to address my long list of ever-growing ailments. Of course, the first thing the nurse wanted me to do was to step on the scale. (Oh Lord: Here we go.) That was always the most devastating part of my visits. This day, I weighed in at around 335 pounds.

When my doctor arrived in the examination room, she reviewed my last blood work results and asked how I was feeling. She commented that she had noticed I had gained more weight. Then, for the first time in about a year-and-a-half, she decided to revisit the subject of weight loss surgery. She asked me once again if I had given it any further thought. She said she had a colleague who was a brilliant weight loss surgeon who could be of help to me.

Once again, I respectfully let her know that I had no interest in weight loss surgery and proceeded to remind her that I had asked her never to bring it up again. Well, what happened next would change my life. My quiet and soft-spoken doctor lifted her head and raised her voice to me! "*Sheila! You will never lose weight on your own! You need help! With your condition, you cannot do this on your own!*" If you have never had a doctor yell at you, let me tell you: It's an eye-opening experience!

Tears rolled from my eyes as I was forced to face my reality. If I was going to have any chance at freedom from my entrapment, I needed help. I wiped my tears and agreed to go to a weight loss surgery seminar. I am so grateful for the tongue-lashing I received from my doctor. She put me in my place and potentially saved my life!

My husband accompanied me to the medical center for the seminar. The room was filled with other overweight and obese people like me, all displaying that undeniable twinkle of hope in their eyes. The surgeons and bariatric staff showed slides and explained three different weight loss surgery options in detail. We were given informational brochures and allowed to ask questions. The staff also permitted us to meet with them individually afterward. The seminar was very informative and dispelled many of the preconceived thoughts I had about the procedures.

With my thyroid issues, I was still not entirely convinced that the surgical option would help me, but I had tried pretty much everything else. In my desperation, I once even thought about using an illegal drug to promote my weight loss. I knew someone who was using a recreational drug and lost weight as a side effect of its use. Even though I do not think I would have ever done it, the mere fact that "Sheila-Do-Right" even *thought* about it was too much. For me, to be so desperate as to even *think* about such a thing was scary. After prayer and meditation, I chose to move forward with the surgery. Even though it was my decision, thankfully my husband rendered his full support.

I joined the Beaumont Hospital Bariatric Program and was connected with a wonderful staff consisting of a surgeon, nurse, and nutritionist. The program allowed me access to a very nice gym with two trainers available to assist me in reaching my goals. I was put on a special diet and given a psychiatric evaluation to ensure I was mentally ready for this change. I exercised three days a week under supervision and saw the surgeon monthly for evaluation. It was a great feeling to have finally made a move—as opposed to just wishing and hoping. Six months later, after successfully following the bariatric program, I was given an appointment to receive my weight loss surgery date. I was beyond excited that a new life could possibly be on the horizon! Or was it…?

Defining Moment 9: Life-Changing Diagnosis: "The Second Final Straw."

One week before receiving my weight loss surgery date, I began having some very unusual health issues. I awakened early one Saturday morning to the entire right side of my body visibly swollen. I was throbbing with pain. By noon, my right hand was almost as big as a baseball mitt. My arm was so swollen and painful that I could barely lift it. My leg, ankle, and foot were severely aching. Even the right side of my face was swollen, and my jaw hurt. Never in my life had I experienced something of this nature. After the pain grew too much to handle, I went to the emergency room. Several tests were taken, but none of the results indicated a diagnosis or the origin of the problem. I was discharged with pain medication.

Two days later, the issues continued to persist. I went back to the emergency room and had a similar experience. Not having any relief, I reached out to my Primary Care Physician. She instructed me to return to the hospital if my symptoms continued and that she would join me there. The following day, I went back to the hospital where even more tests were performed. The emergency room was very crowded, so I was being examined and treated in the middle of the floor, just a few steps from the nurse's station. The emergency room doctor came to me and casually asked me if anyone had ever told me I had leukemia. I responded that no one had ever mentioned this to me because I did not *have* leukemia. He let me know in clear terms that I did indeed show all the signs of having this rare bone and blood cancer called Chronic Myeloid Leukemia or "CML."

Instead of being shocked, I was in a form of denial. I honestly assumed there had been a mix-up in the emergency room or maybe even a fluke in the blood test results. I had minimal worries. I was admitted to the hospital. My doctor arrived and worked alongside the emergency room physicians. I spent several days in the hospital being tested and examined.

In order to get conclusive results, I needed to be given a bone marrow biopsy. Once again, my obesity made it very difficult to administer the test. A common location for a bone marrow aspiration is the rear upper pelvic bone. Unfortunately, since my rear was so huge and fatty, the doctors literally had their hands full trying to get a proper sample. The first attempt was unsuccessful and had to be tried again the following day. The second attempt was successful, and the bone marrow was sent for testing.

After six days of being poked and prodded, I was sent home and given a doctor's appointment for further treatment. Even though I was told that all signs pointed to me having cancer, I was in denial and borderline unfazed. I was more concerned that I had missed my appointment to get my weight loss surgery date. I wanted to get home, call my bariatric doctor, and reschedule my appointment to get **"unfat."** I am still flabbergasted that the thought of being obese initially scared me more than the thought of having cancer.

The Monday after returning home from my hospital stay, I went to see my Primary Care Physician for final test results and a follow-up. Typically, when I went to her office, I was directed into either Exam Room 2 or 3. However, this time I was ushered into Exam Room 1. I thought it was odd that I had never been placed in this room. We would always walk past it on the way to one of the other rooms. Exam Room 1 looked nothing like the other exam rooms. It looked like a small lounge area. This room had plush seating, soft lighting, and soothing décor. The nurse offered me a seat, and I waited for the doctor to enter. As I waited, I wondered why I had never been in this room. Instantly it hit me: This was the bad news room! This was the place where sad test results were given.

My doctor came in and verified my suspicions. She confirmed that the bone marrow biopsy did indeed show that I had CML. My doctor had a look of concern in her eyes unlike one I had ever seen. I needed to know if there was more to this story. I wanted to know the average life expectancy of people with this disease. My doctor said that I needed to consult a specialist on the matter. I persisted and again asked her, "To your knowledge, what is the average life expectancy?" I was told five years. She reiterated this was not her specialty and that the information needed to be discussed and confirmed with an oncologist.

"...but all I heard was **five years**."

At that moment, my life seemed to stand still. It was like a dark cloud rested above my head and followed me. I left the doctor's office with my paperwork and information for an oncologist appointment. From the medical center parking lot, I called my husband and told him that **I had cancer**—

CANCER! He offered to come to the doctor's office to drive me home, but I declined. I needed to be alone, if only for a while. My drive home is still a vague memory. I have no recollection of being in traffic. It was as though I was teleported from the doctor's office to my driveway. I was in a complete haze.

My faith was again being tested. I wanted to believe that this was not happening or that I would be healed. Instead, I went full-throttle into a pity party. "Why me Lord? Haven't I lived a life pleasing in Your sight? I may not be perfect, but haven't I dedicated my life to Kingdom work?" This was not fair! All I could think about was how would I explain this to my children and grandchildren. I loved my children more than life itself and did not want them to experience any pain. My mind was zooming with all the things I needed to accomplish within the years before my impending demise.

Thank God for intercessors. My remarkable husband stepped in and became my spiritual mediator. He prayed and fasted on my behalf while I constantly cried and Googled everything I could find out about the disease. Instead of praying as I should have, I was on the internet searching for a ray of hope. I cried and Googled, then I Googled and cried. I have always loved my husband, but my love for him grew to another level. While I was wallowing in my humanness, God gave my amazing, selfless husband the sense to pray and fast *for* me.

After two weeks of crying and extreme sadness, I met with an oncologist. She let me know that years ago, it was true that the average life expectancy for CML was about five years. Thankfully, new treatments were available, and most people now lived their full life expectancy! She said that I *would* die one day, but it probably would not be from CML! I cannot express how happy I was to hear those words!

A few weeks later, I began an oral chemotherapy treatment. I was instructed to take the chemotherapy twice daily. The initial treatment was intense and came with some unpleasant side effects, but I considered it a huge blessing! My daily oral chemo was a fair trade-off for my life. I am grateful to God, my incredible husband, and all the others who stood in the gap and prayed for me when I could not seem to pray for myself.

Once I knew that I would live, I asked my oncologist if I was allowed to go ahead with weight loss surgery. She let me know that we could not move forward at that time because my response to treatment needed to be monitored closely. Additionally, there was not a lot of data that indicated how well the chemo medication would be absorbed in a smaller stomach like those of weight loss surgery patients. Meanwhile, weight loss surgery was put on the back burner—and rightfully so.

She let me know that we could revisit the subject in a year. One year later, I excitedly brought up weight loss surgery to my oncologist. My chemo treatment was going well, so I hoped we could move forward. The response again was, "No. We will revisit the subject in another year." I could not argue my case. I needed my oncologist to be completely secure and confident about allowing me to proceed. Meanwhile, unlike others with cancer who lost weight, I continued to gain.

Finally, in early 2014 my oncologist shared that the treatment response of my red and white blood cells was going very well I was released to explore weight loss surgery. Of course, I was ecstatic! Unfortunately, by then my health insurance had changed, and I was no longer able to resume my position at the Beaumont Bariatric Program. I now had to go to the Henry Ford Hospital Bariatric Program and start the process all over again! It was a program that lasted about nine months! I was devastated. I began to question if it was even meant to be.

Every time I tried to move forward one step, I seemingly ended up taking several steps backward. I was extremely discouraged. After thought and prayer, I concluded that if I quit on myself, I would stay trapped in my pain. I began to encourage myself. I convinced myself to make a move and that it would all be worth it in the long run. I joined the program and then researched and selected a surgeon.

At the initial appointment, I weighed in at an embarrassing 346 pounds and was told I needed to lose 15 pounds before surgery. I was assigned a bariatric nurse, a nutritionist, and attended support groups and informational classes. I followed the diet and instructions in the informational binder that I was given. It was very challenging for me with my slow metabolism, but over a few months, I managed to slowly lose the 15 pounds.

I was doing well until tragedy struck. My family suffered the loss of three family members within a few weeks. We were all devastated. In my distraction, I put my nutritional guidelines on the back burner. In October 2014, I had an appointment to receive my surgery date. I was very excited! The nurse weighed me, and the number on the scale was not in my favor. I had regained 7 of the 15 pounds I lost.

My doctor told me that due to the weight regain, my surgery would be postponed until I gained control of my habits and lost the weight again. I was beyond hurt! I explained to him that I was distracted by life's challenges and told him about all the funerals I had just attended. He then shared with me that life will always have its challenges. He stated that challenges should never be an excuse for me to not take care of myself. My surgeon reminded me that I could not control what happens to others and that I needed to maintain control of my own health and welfare.

Even though I knew he was right, I was fuming. I left the doctor's office in tears. Here is yet another hurdle for me to jump over. The doctor's receptionist gave me a follow-up appointment for the following year! I couldn't come back until February 2015! As angry as I was, I had done this to myself. There was no one else to blame. I was crushed. Clearly, I was meant to stay fat.

During those four months, I learned a valuable lesson. I already knew that weight retention was a symptom of my hypothyroidism. It was clear that losing weight would always be very difficult for me. It finally clicked that I needed to work harder for what I wanted; perhaps even harder than others. I learned that no part of this journey was going to come easy for me. I was going to have to FIGHT! Doing nothing was not an option. Wallowing in self-pity was not an option. Blaming life's circumstances was not an option. If I wanted freedom from my entrapment, it was up to me to *believe* that "I could do all things through Christ that strengthened me!" Even though I could not control everything regarding my body and health, I knew I needed to change whatever I *could*.

"*Change happens when the pain of staying the same is greater than the pain of change.*" This quote by Tony Robbins resonates with me in a powerful way. Life definitely deals us challenging hands, but we have the choice whether to accept or reject them and push through. The pain in which I was trapped finally outweighed any possible pain I could endure by making a change. It took me a while to embrace the level of change I needed to save my life, but I got there. The fact that I awakened is far more important than how many wake-up calls it took. Woke is woke. Fully awake, I asked God to strengthen me so I could do the things I needed to do!

I resumed the diet given to me from the bariatric center. The bone pain as a result of my cancer and chemo treatment was quite intense. My feet and joints hurt horribly from the excess weight I carried. Still, I continued to push myself to exercise at my gym three days a week. Many days I worked out in pain and in tears.

The experience with my bariatric surgeon had been eye-opening. It was unpleasant, but it had also given me a fresh determination to succeed. I felt challenged and decided to accept the challenge. I returned to my doctor in February 2015. I had lost the weight and was given a date that I now affectionately refer to as my "Second Birthdate": April 20, 2015 — my weight loss surgery date!

"Three people may travel three different roads to get to the same destination. Their routes and methods of travel may differ; but if they stay the course, they will all arrive at the same endpoint. Just find the route that is best for you and travel."

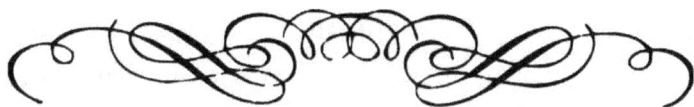

Chapter 6

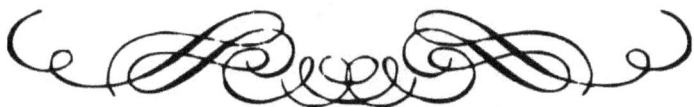

Weight Loss Surgery: My Life-Saving Tool

Finally, all of my defining moments had a purpose. My experiences may have been painful, but they drove me to change. I knew that the route I chose to save my life was drastic, but the operative word for me was *save* — not drastic. This is a decision in which I am not ashamed, and I will never apologize for making this choice.

On April 20, 2015, I checked into the hospital surgery center at 7:30 a.m. to prepare for gastric sleeve surgery. With this procedure, part of my stomach would be removed and then the surgeon would join the remaining portions together to make a new banana-sized stomach or "sleeve." This would allow me to feel full quicker and help me lose weight. Additionally, this surgery removes the part of your stomach that makes a hormone that boosts your appetite, so for a few months, many cravings decrease or even dissipate.

It was explained to me that there was a "honeymoon" phase with weight loss surgery. I could expect to lose the majority of weight during the first few months' post-operative. It was my job to encourage this loss with proper nutrition, vitamins, and regular exercise. It was also made clear to me that a new healthy lifestyle and habits were mandatory for maintenance of the weight loss.

I was a bundle of nerves, but more excited than scared. I was ready. The risks were minimal but still present. I understood this, but I was strong in my *faith* and had followed up with my *works*. I had gone through the pre-surgical, 2-week liquid diet with a breeze. The liquid diet was designed to shrink my liver, making the surgical process easier. Now, I was ready to take on a new lifestyle.

My surgery was a success! When I awakened in recovery, I pulled my covers back and joked with my surgeon and his team: "Oh Lord, my surgery didn't take. I'm still fat!" With this exhibited sense of humor, they—and I—knew I was just fine. I experienced the typical gas, soreness, and nausea associated with this procedure, but no complications.

I went home armed with my new tool for success. I had paid attention to what was taught in bariatric class and referred to my informational binder often. I did not want to fail yet again. However, I was still quite skeptical. Honestly, I was just not positive the procedure would even work for me due to my hypothyroidism. But when I went to my first post-op doctor's appointment, I was already down 20 pounds!

As soon as my physician released me, which was at ten weeks out, I resumed my workout regimen. I started simply with walking, graduated to speed walking, and then began high incline walking. Eventually, I began to run! The day I ran on the treadmill, I burst into tears. I had lost about 50 pounds so far and could hardly believe that the same person who could barely walk was now running! My motivation grew more and more as I saw results.

I increased my workouts to 4 to 6 days a week. I had always enjoyed exercise, but my love was growing even more. I stayed true to my diet provided to me by my nutritionist. By the time I was five months out, I was down 70 pounds. I had very little desire to cheat on my diet or go back to my old ways. My new habits were working for me. My former habits were not, so it did not make sense for me to go backward. Forward was the only way to go.

At 18 months post-op, I was a full-blown fitness junkie and had lost a whopping 146 pounds! In December 2016, I finally reach the coveted and ever-popular "ONEderland" — a number on the scale that begins with *one*. My scale reflected 197 pounds. As a 51-year-old, I wept with joy to see a number I had not seen since I was 21-years old!

Many asked how I was so successful during this process. I like to use my Lawnmower Analogy. When you buy a home, you need to cut your grass, so you buy a lawnmower. You can just set your mower in the middle of the yard, and yes, it will automatically cut a little grass even if you do nothing else. Now, for maximum results, you've got to push it! Walk with it! Work it! You need to gas it up, change the oil, and keep it properly maintained. Your lawn will be immaculate with a well-tuned machine! Having this tool is an incredible blessing, but if you do not work it, you cannot maximize its benefits.

"Real change starts with your thoughts. Your body will go where your mind takes you."

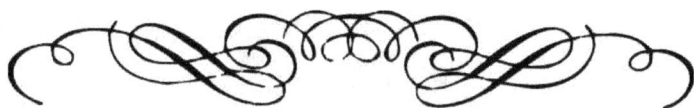

Chapter 7

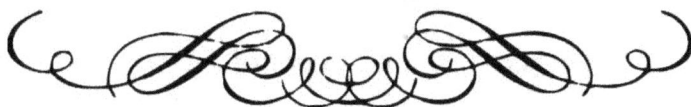

Change Your Mindset

How you think and how you handle your thoughts has a direct relation to what you eat and what you do with your body. I have learned that for optimal success, a change in your mindset is mandatory. Create a permanent shift in your attitude. Drop bad habits and replace them with better ones. Decide what you want and where you want to go, and then devise a plan to get there. It all starts with a thought. Perform your research and study until it resonates.

Tailor your plan to what motivates you, and you will have a better chance at being successful. What moves you toward pleasure and away from pain is what is perceived. I decided to reprogram my mind to look at exercise as pleasurable and junk food as painful. This is a simple trick, but it works!

My Primary Care Physician told me to look at fattening foods as if I am allergic to them. Now, I know I am not "allergic" to potato chips in the traditional way, but when I am tempted to eat too many of them or something else that I know I should avoid, I remind myself that I will have an allergic reaction (weight gain) if I consume it. It works for me! Use whatever "trick" necessary to change your mindset!

Find or create a visual motivational tool. I constructed a vision board that displayed many of the things I desired to do, see, or become. My vision board has several pictures regarding weight loss, beating cancer, and writing a book. I placed the board on the side of my bed so it would be in my face. Looking at the board helped me engrain these desires in my mind. I am now walking in those visions.

"Short-term goals lead to long-term successes. Write them down and then realize them. Consistency is the key."

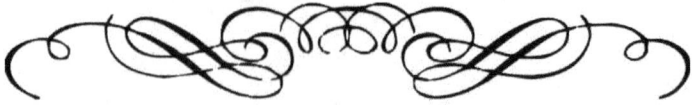

Chapter 8

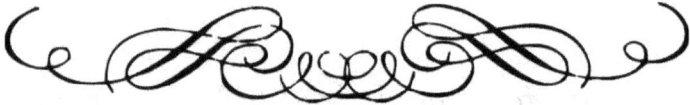

Short-Term Goals

Write down your short-term goals. Then, consider the challenges associated with reaching them and ask yourself: Where will I be in one year (five years, etc.) if I continue with unhealthy lifestyle choices? Find the pain in undesirable choices. Make these associations connect with *pain*.

Then, write down long-term desires and benefits of healthy lifestyle choices. Ask yourself where you will be in the future if you incorporate these positive choices (for example; live longer, be an inspiration to others, be around to see your grandchildren grow up, etc.). Find pleasure in desirable and healthy choices. Make these associations connect with *joy*.

Start building good habits. Continue them until they become second-nature. Program yourself by making healthy eating and exercise habits. Set small, 30-day challenges with things you know you can do. Then, once they become a habit or too easy, add to or increase the challenge and/or length of time. Give yourself one full month to allow a new behavior to become habitual, thereby decreasing the chances of falling back into old habits.

I have found that gradual changes work best. I trained my mind to accept a new behavior as the norm. In the beginning, consistency is more important than quantity. Practice some type of new behavior daily until it feels normal and natural. "I enjoy _____!" Fill in the blank with what you know you can do. But don't be afraid to try something new. In my quest to become physically fit, I have tried the trampoline workout, treadmill, HIIT workout, kickboxing, jogging and running, bicycling, roller skating, and weightlifting. I have found that it is good to start with small steps and then build endurance over time. This creates lasting motivation.

I set a realistic weight loss goal for myself. I knew that I wanted to lose a total of 175 pounds, but when I looked at the huge number, I got overwhelmed. I knew that it would be difficult for me to celebrate losing 5 pounds if I still had "…with 170 pounds to go" still looking at me in my face. Every inch and every pound lost is worthy of celebration.

I decided to break it down to three achievable increments. My first goal was to get out of the 300s. I was thrilled the day I saw 298 on my scale. My second goal was to achieve a 100-pound weight loss. My third goal was to reach "ONEderland." Every few months, I was able to check one of these goals off my list and move to the next. The feeling was exhilarating. Even while enduring many weight loss stalls, having clear, short-term goals allowed me to remain focused, encouraged, and kept anxiety at bay.

"My body is my personal gift from God. How I treat it shows my level of appreciation for this gift."

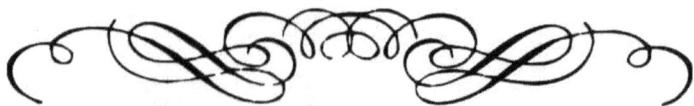

Chapter 9

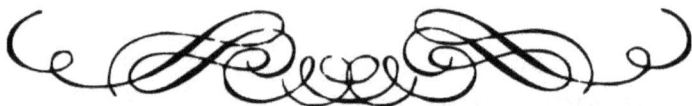

Proper Nutrition

As I am not a medical professional, I strongly recommended getting a meal plan from a licensed dietician or nutritionist. Generally speaking, most bariatric patients consume 900 to 1,000 calories, 64 ounces of water, and at least 60 to 80 grams of protein daily. Typical meals include low-fat dairy products, lean cuts of beef, chicken, pork, or fish, beans, nuts, vegetables, and eggs—just to name a few. These are good protein sources. Foods that are high in sugar and fat should be avoided after weight loss surgery, as it may be difficult for your digestive system to tolerate those particular foods.

What has been very beneficial to me was closely tracking my protein, water, and calorie intake. My first year after surgery, I tracked my intake "TO THE LETTER." I tracked it until it became second-nature. There are wonderful apps available, but I went old-school: I used a writing tablet. I made up a chart and filled it out all day as I ate and drank. Initially, the columns were Protein (60-80) / Water (64) / Calories (850-1000), and then Breakfast / Lunch / Snacks. Meal prepping was a life-saver. I prepared and packed all of my meals and snacks according to my guidelines.

To stay on track, I ate only what I prepared and rarely diverted. I was *super-strict* on myself. My sacrifice paid off and eventually even stopped feeling like a sacrifice. I enjoyed my new diet. My bariatric nutritionist devised my diet plan. I was closely monitored. Again, for optimal success, a specific diet and instructions should come from your medical professional.

"Make moves — and then stop stopping!"

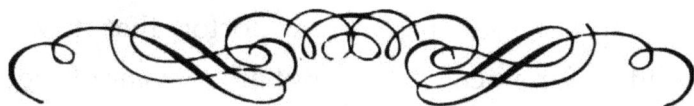

Chapter 10

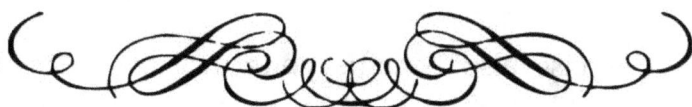

Move It to Lose It - Exercise

My first-year post-op, I worked out 4 to 6 days a week. I have always enjoyed working out, but it was challenging due to the bone and joint pain. Thankfully, my pain level has decreased drastically, and exercise is actually fun for me now.

Since there was a time that exercise was very painful for me, I now embrace the opportunity to work out. In fact, I find it a privilege. There are so many benefits to exercise. Both cardio and weight-training have health benefits. It burns calories that lead to weight loss. Exercise lowers your risk for many diseases, including heart disease and obesity.

Years ago, I was told by a doctor that I was a candidate for a heart attack. But after a year of regular exercise, my oncologist told me that I now have the heart rate of an athlete! This meant a great deal to me. Weight loss leads to better health, but exercise leads to fitness.

Exercise also benefits your mental health. It releases endorphins in your brain that relieve stress and pain, and also decreases fatigue. An endorphin release produces an attitude that is positive—even euphoric. I can go into the gym tired and leave out energized!

Working out was and still is important to me—not just for weight loss, but also for overall health and fitness. I prefer to work out 1-2 hours at a time. As to not get bored, I mix things up. I walk, run, and weight-train. I find many fun and interesting routines on YouTube.

While I prefer working out at a gym, I also run at the park and do exercise routines at home if I cannot make it outdoors. I purchased a yoga mat, resistance bands, dumbbells, and kettlebells. Having equipment at home ensures I can maximize my workout and also leaves me with no excuses for missing a workout. I love to work out until I drip in sweat as fat is expelled through the lungs, urine, and perspiration.

I believe that in order to lose it (weight), I have to move it (my body)! Figure out what works for you and get moving. Just stop stopping! Remain consistent and diligent, and you will see results. I embrace a "Zero Excuses" mentality. My goal was to transform my body and my life. Working out has taught me that with discipline, I can do just that. I transformed! It is an amazing feeling to now love even the reflection of myself. My outside is now matching what I felt on the inside.

"Faith without works is dead.
Period."

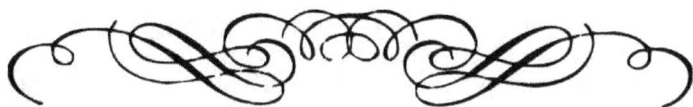

Chapter 11

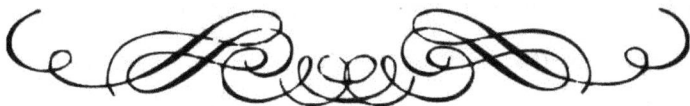

The Soul Connection - Prayer

Connect with God for strength and guidance. Philippians 4:13 says: *"I can do all things through Christ that strengthens me."* Believe that! Trust God's Word and know in your heart that it is true. Know that "His Word will never return unto Him void." My faith was indeed tested, and I had many moments when I felt I would be trapped in my morbid obesity forever. Even though there were moments when I struggled, I continued to exercise my faith.

I encourage you also to exercise your faith! Start to see yourself as you want to be, then put a plan into action and make it come to fruition. Remember:

"Faith without works is dead." You have to *do* something. You have to make a move! God has made provisions for us to live life more abundantly. It is our choice whether to embrace what He has provided or not. Just as we have free-will in our choice to believe in and live for God, we also have the choice to live a clean and healthy life right here on earth. Our bodies are temples—our own personal gifts from God.

I have learned (and am still learning) to honor my temple (my body) in my actions by how I treat and feed it. I have found that in being better fit, I am not only benefitting my natural life, but I am also more effective in the Kingdom work and my personal worship. 1 Corinthians 6:19-20 (NIV) says, *"Do you not know that your bodies are temples of the Holy Spirit, who is in you, whom you have received from God? You are not your own; you were bought at a price."*

Therefore, honor God with your body. Having a relationship with The Creator gives us the strength to endure and even overcome many of life's challenges. We are empowered to withstand obstacles and push towards our life's goals. God wants our lives on this earth to be prosperous and happy. It is up to us to take the gift that He gave us and use it for His will and His glory. We must treat it as the gift that it is.

Make exercise and movement purposeful and fun. Focus on things you enjoy doing versus things you find boring or mundane. Focus on healthy foods you enjoy and eat those. God placed some awesome foods and activities within our reach that are not only beneficial but enjoyable. Find them and incorporate them into your life.

It is popular and even normal to speak life. Speak energy into and about the things you want. I have learned to tell myself that I will succeed rather than wallowing in self-pity. I speak the things that I want God to bless me with. I started calling myself a writer before I was published. I spoke life into the words that I wanted to share with others who may be at a crossroad.

Conversely, there comes an occasion where speaking death comes into play. Speaking death is also a verbal and articulated act of faith. The same way you speak something into existence is the same way you speak to the demise of an unhealthy issue. I learned to speak death to my cancer. It is now almost undetectable! I spoke death to my obesity. I am no longer obese! Speak death to the things in your life that are not of God.

Speaking the ruin of negative things is an active show of confidence and assurance that you refuse to accept the undesired. Whether spiritual or physical, I have learned to speak death and openly rebuke things that hinder my growth. Therefore, I speak death to cancer, obesity, sickness, negativity, and toxic relationships. I speak death to anything that does not encourage or progress my journey.

"People who criticize are toxic.
They will anger, discourage, and
plant seeds of negativity."

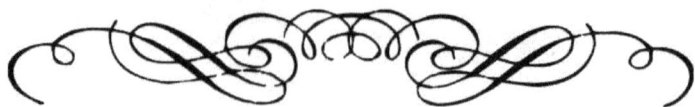

Chapter 12

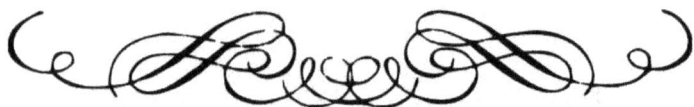

Find Support

It is much easier to stick with a weight loss plan when you have support. Surround yourself with people who support your healthy changes. Look for a friend that can share tips on diet and exercise. People who criticize are toxic and will anger, discourage, and plant seeds of negativity. I work out well alone, as it helps me to stay focused. Many people are motivated to work out with a buddy. Find a friend who will encourage you. You will motivate each other.

Look at all options! Social media has many active support groups dedicated to weight loss, health, and fitness. I belong to a few online groups that are specifically catered to bariatric weight loss. I also joined several groups that focus on weightlifting, juicing, and vegetarian diets. I have obtained a wealth of knowledge from these groups, and the friendships made have been invaluable.

Hospitals, universities, and medical centers have groups that meet to support and motivate. They are platforms that allow you to vent and share both your challenges and your victories. These groups are facilitated by psychologists, nutritionists, and other weight loss professionals. This is a huge asset.

Gyms and fitness centers also have classes dedicated to fitness and wellness. In joining classes, you can meet other like-minded people for support. They can help you stay on track while on your health and wellness journey.

Just because you are not busy
does not mean that you are available.
Guard your time!

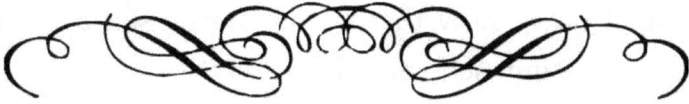

Chapter 13

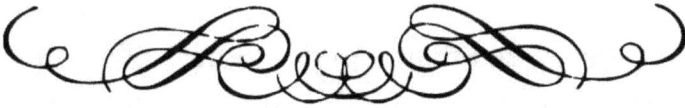

Make Yourself a Priority

I have learned that no one can make me a priority in the way that I can. Unapologetically, I devoted much of my youth and time to the care of my children and home. Now, the door has been opened for me to provide myself with a greater level of self-care and love. Initially, I experienced some feelings of guilt in making myself a priority. I had become accustomed to looking out for others and neglecting myself. I love helping others. Being in a position to help others is a blessing. My family will always be the most important thing in my life. I also realize that if I do not take care of myself, I will not be any good for them. I now know that in making myself a priority and exercising self-care, I can better show love to them. The old, obese, broken down version of myself could only provide limited service to my family. Not only did my trapped situation provide a disservice to myself; it also provided a disservice to my family.

I discovered that I am deserving of "me-time." Even if it's just a 30-minute walk in the park, I deserve to take this time. After all, if everyone else around me is worthy of care and attention, so am I! Just because you are not busy does not mean you are available. Guard your time! You not only deserve your time; you need it. It is a wonderful thing to be available for others, but if you do not prioritize and make time for yourself, it will leave you frustrated and overwhelmed. Loving yourself will better equip you to love others.

Making the decision to have weight loss surgery required me to make myself a priority. For various reasons, people may try to talk you out of doing what is best for you. Regardless of the opinions of others, I chose to make saving my life a priority.

"Despite life's ups and downs, I find it important to just keep it moving. There's growth in movement."

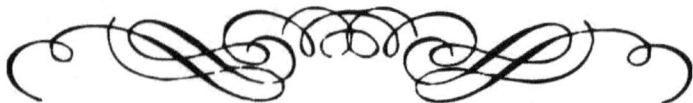

Chapter 14

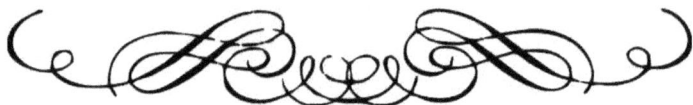

Final Thoughts

I feel blessed to share my testimony. I do so with the desire to inspire hope. Despite the many obstacles the adversary put in my way to deter me, I chose not to let them stop me from making moves. I chose not to let my obstacles be my excuses. Instead, my obstacles were my inspiration! They *were* my reasons for moving forward. Life is full of obstacles, including people who try to talk you out of doing what is best for you. Regardless of naysayers, you must move forward.

The route I took to lead myself out of morbid obesity is not the route for everyone. The decision was very personal. What I want to convey is that whatever path you decide to take to better your health, just make a move! It does not have to involve surgery; just change! Do something different! Be your own motivation, even when others are not encouraging you. It all starts in the mind. Real change begins with your thoughts. Your body will go where your minds takes you.

Weight loss surgery (gastric sleeve) is the tool I used to help me *get* the weight off. Proper diet and consistent exercise are the tools I use to help me *keep* the weight off. The "magic" of weight loss surgery is not permanent. My body has adjusted to the smaller food portions; therefore, in order to achieve long-term or permanent success, new habits needed to be formed and adhered to permanently. In conjunction with my hypothyroidism, the return to former habits will more than likely put me back on the road to obesity. This process requires an actual lifestyle change. Whether your obesity was brought on from a medical condition, food addiction, or emotional eating, the root has to be identified and then dealt with or else it is sure to resurface.

This process has been a blessing to me in so many ways. Not only has my weight loss led to better health, but it has also increased my self-confidence. Once I began to practice self-care, the more I cared. I have a brand-new quality of life! I have gone from barely being able to walk to running. I have completed four 5Ks to date, which is still mind-blowing to me! I used to hide, but I was honored to walk the runway in a fashion show — and it was exhilarating! Initially a journalism major and student writer, I finally found the courage to apply for a writer's position at a local paper and have been writing for them for over a year.

Despite how shy I was with regards to standing in front of people, I stepped out on faith and launched what (hopefully) is the beginning of an acting career. So far, I've have acted in four stage plays and just accepted my first role in a film! No, weight loss did not make all of this happen, but as I began to work on improving my body and health, it inspired me to improve other areas of life as well. In my 50's, it was not too late for me to change my life.

Despite life's ups and downs, I find it important to just keep it moving. There's growth in movement. As painful as some of my experiences were, I now know that they were assigned to me because I could handle them without breaking. I also know that despite the tears, tantrums, health challenges, judgment, embarrassment, and sadness, that entrapment was assigned to me. At times I may have *bent*, but thanks to God's grace and mercy, I did not break.

Some folks say that opting for weight loss surgery is the "easy way out." I have since made an interesting observation. People with other medical conditions seek out help, and no one seems to talk them out of doing what is best for their health. If I had a tumor, whether benign or cancerous, and my physician recommended that it be removed to avoid possible future complications, most people would support my decision to have it removed.

Even if I had something much more minor like a mole in the center of my forehead and sought medical attention to get it removed, most people would say, "Yes, if it's bothering you, go ahead and handle it." However, for some reason, if you seek surgical attention for obesity, it is shunned and thought of as cheating. I believe there is more than one way to reach a goal. The route to a destination will never be identical for everyone, and that is okay.

This process is certainly not easy. However, if people want to continue to say it is the easy way out, let them say it! For me, it was easier than remaining in pain. It was easier than letting my health issues continue to mount. It was easier than continuing to diminish my quality of life. It was easier than dying an early death. So, if weight loss surgery was the easy way out, I'm glad I took it! I am no longer trapped. I am free and alive to tell my story!

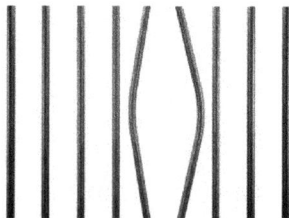

References

Bible Gateway (2018) Online Bible (NKJV). Retrieved from https://wwwbiblegatewaycom

ClipArtBest.com

Cohen, R, (2014) As U S waistlines expand, seatbelt use falls Retrieved from https//www.reuters.com

Breast Cancer Facts: Ethnicity & Race. Retrieved from https://my.clevelandclinic.org

Webster, M, (2018) Dictionary. Retrieved from https://wwwmerriamwebstercom

Tootsie Roll Inc. (2018) Tootsie Roll Industries Retrieved from https://wwwtootsiecom

www.ingramcontent.com/pod-product-compliance
Lightning Source LLC
Chambersburg PA
CBHW071231290326
41931CB00037B/2678